Basic Audiometry

FREDERICK N. MARTIN

5341 Industrial Oaks Boulevard
Austin, Texas 78735

**The PRO-ED
studies in
communicative disorders**

Series editor
HARVEY HALPERN

Copyright © 1986 by PRO-ED, Inc.
Printed in the United States of America.
All rights reserved. No part of this book may be reproduced in any form or
by any means without the prior written permission of the publisher.

Library of Congress Cataloging in Publication Data
Martin, Frederick N.
  Basic audiometry.

  (The Pro-Ed studies in communicative disorders)
  Bibliography: p.
  1. Audiometry. I. Title. II. Series. [DNLM: 1. Audiometry. WV 272
M379b]
RF294.M368   1986   617.8'075   86-9376
ISBN 0-89079-084-1

5341 Industrial Oaks Boulevard
Austin, Texas 78735

        10 9 8 7 6 5 4 3 2 1   86 87 88 89 90 91

Contents

Preface

Since its inception four decades ago, the science of audiology has changed rapidly. Modern technological advances have dramatically altered the kinds of equipment that audiologists use, but equipment is only as good as the clinicians who use it for the betterment of their patients. While audiometric testing is only one small part of audiological management of hearing-impaired persons, it is essential that diagnostic tests be carried out accurately and that results be appropriately interpreted. This monograph introduces the reader to the basic principles of hearing testing, including pure-tone audiometry, speech audiometry, and immittance measures.

Basic Audiometry

Introduction

In the days predating the electronic era, people's interest in disorders of hearing led to the development of a number of tests of hearing sensitivity. These ranged from the use of a variety of noisemakers creating loud sounds, to the soft click of two coins, to the more sophisticated tuning-fork tests.

Hearing can be tested in two general ways: air conduction and bone conduction. Sounds heard by air conduction are those that enter the outer ear, are propagated through the middle ear, transduced into electrical impulses in the inner ear, and conducted along the auditory nerve to the brainstem and then, via various relay stations, to the auditory cortex. Sounds heard by bone conduction are those which have enough energy to vibrate the skull, thereby setting the fluids of the inner ear into vibration and stimulating the hair cells of the cochlea. Other mechanisms contribute to our hearing by bone conduction, but they are beyond the intent of this monograph and are well covered elsewhere (Dirks, 1985). The outer and middle ears are generally considered to be the conductive apparatus for hearing, and the cochlea and retrocochlear structures the sensorineural mechanisms.

Obviously, a person having no difficulty in any of the anatomical loci named above has normal hearing and hears sounds well by both air and bone conduction. A patient with a sensorineural loss of hearing has difficulty hearing by both air and bone conduction, and a patient with a conductive hearing loss has some depression of hearing by air conduction with normal bone conduction.

Tuning-Fork Tests

Tuning forks are instruments made of magnesium alloy on steel that are designed, when activated, to vibrate at particular frequencies, usually corresponding closely with the musical scale of C.

While audiologists rarely conduct tuning-fork tests, these tests should be reviewed both from a historical and an academic point of view. The three most commonly performed tuning-fork tests are the Schwabach, the Rinne, and the Weber. Two other valuable but less frequently used tuning-fork tests are the Bing and Gelle tests.

The Schwabach Test

This test was designed to compare the hearing by bone conduction of a patient with that of the examiner. After the fork has been set into vibration by striking it against a firm but resilient surface (the heel of the shoe does well for this purpose, as a more solid surface may damage the fork and alter its frequency), the stem of the fork is placed on the mastoid process of the patient. The patient is instructed to indicate when the tone is heard. The fork is then alternately placed on the mastoid of the patient and the examiner as the amplitude decays until neither hears the tone. The Schwabach test indicates whether the patient and examiner hear the tone for the same length of time (normal Schwabach), whether the patient hears the tone for a shorter time than the examiner (shortened Schwabach), or whether the patient hears the tone longer than the examiner (prolonged Schwabach).

The Schwabach test is interpreted as follows. When patients hear the tone for the same period of time as the examiner, their hearing (for the tested frequency and for bone conduction only) is normal—that is, if the examiner's hearing is normal. The patient with a prolonged Schwabach is said to have a conductive impairment, and the patient with a shortened Schwabach, a sensorineural loss of hearing. While the Schwabach test is easy to perform, it is just as easy to misinterpret. Information is gained only at the frequency tested, and the examiner may not have normal hearing for this frequency. In addition, it may be fallacious to assume that the ear being tested is on the same side of the head as the tuning fork, as it is quite easy for bone-conduction vibrations to lateralize (travel) to the opposite ear. The proper position for the tuning fork when performing the Schwabach test is shown in Figure 1A (Pappas, Bailey, & Martin, 1966).

The Rinne Test

This test is designed to compare patients' hearing by air conduction (Figure 1B) with their hearing by bone conduction (Figure 1A). There are probably more

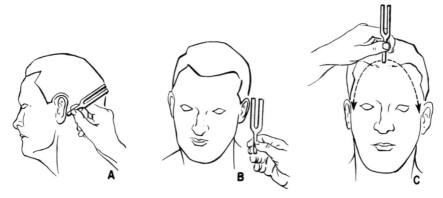

Figure 1.   Positions for tuning-fork tests. From Pappas, Bailey, and Martin (1966). Reprinted by permission.

individual variations on this test than on any other tuning-fork test. The way the Rinne test is usually performed is to ask the patient whether the tone is louder by air or bone conduction. Since air conduction is a more efficient means of sound transmission, the patient with normal hearing for the frequency tested will hear the signal louder with the tines of the fork held next to the ear than with the stem held against the mastoid process. This is called a positive Rinne. A positive Rinne is also found in cases with sensorineural hearing loss. Patients with conductive loss will hear the tone louder behind the ear than at the ear since their problem is in the conductive mechanism of the outer and/or middle ear. This is called a negative Rinne. Some persons with mild conductive losses show positive Rinne results. Usually a conductive loss of more than about 25 decibels is required to offset the normal superiority of air conduction over bone conduction.

In addition to the common problems in remembering which test is negative and which is positive in this context, the Rinne test presents the problem of the "false negative." A patient with poor bone conduction in one ear will hear the tone louder by bone conduction in the contralateral ear (if that ear has better bone conduction) than by air conduction in the test ear. This may lead examiners to think they are dealing with a conductive rather than a sensorineural loss.

The Weber Test

This test is valid only when a unilateral hearing loss is present and is performed by placing the stem of the vibrating fork on the forehead or midline of the patient's head (Figure 1C). The patient is then simply asked to state the ear in which the tone is heard. If the tone is heard (or heard louder) in the better ear, it is assumed that the ear with poorer hearing suffers a sensorineural loss. Conversely, if the tone lateralizes to the poorer-hearing ear, it is suggestive of a conductive loss in that ear.

The reason for the tone being heard in the better ear in unilateral sensorineural loss is understandable on the basis of the Stenger principle. The Stenger principle states that if two tones of the same frequency are introduced simultaneously into both ears, only the louder one is perceived. Obviously, the impaired bone conduction of the poorer ear attenuates the signal (decreases the loudness) so that it is stronger in the better ear. A number of explanations for the lateralization to the poorer ear in a unilateral conductive loss have been advanced, but none has been proved conclusively.

The Weber test may be misleading in several ways. Some persons with unilateral conductive hearing losses are reluctant to report that they hear the sound louder in the ear that they know to be poorer. In addition, the patient with a long-standing hearing loss in one ear may not have an appreciation of the "rightness" or "leftness" of a signal.

The Bing Test

In the performance of the Bing test the stem of the tuning fork with the tines vibrating is placed on the mastoid process of the patient (Figure 1A). The examiner then alternately occludes and unoccludes the opening into the external auditory meatus by pushing a finger into the canal or by pressing the tragus into the canal. When patients continue to hear a steady tone, the conclusion is that they have a conductive loss at this frequency. If the tone appears to pulsate or change in loudness, this means that they have normal hearing or a sensorineural hearing loss at the test frequency.

Because of the often-studied but not entirely understood "occlusion effect," closing off the opening of the external auditory canal will cause an increase in the subjective loudness of bone-conducted tones unless the patient has a conductive hearing loss. Most patients with conductive losses do not manifest the occlusion effect. Since the occlusion effect occurs primarily in the low frequencies, this test is not applicable for tones above 1000 Hz.

The Gelle Test

Of all tuning-fork tests the Gelle is the most difficult to perform and easiest to misinterpret. It is based upon the principle of centripetal pressure, comparing the effects of positive air pressure in the external auditory canal on tonal loud-

TABLE 1
Interpretation of Tuning-Fork Tests

Test	Normal Hearing	Conductive Loss	Sensorineural Loss
Schwabach	Normal	Prolonged or normal	Shortened
Rinne	Positive	Negative	Positive
Weber	Does not lateralize	Lateralizes to poorer ear	Lateralizes to better ear
Bing	Tone pulsates	Tone remains steady	Tone pulsates
Gelle	Decreases sensitivity for air conduction and bone conduction	Decreases sensitivity for air conduction; bone conduction unchanged	Decreases sensitivity for air conduction and bone conduction

ness. This test requires the use of a tuning fork with a frequency not above 1000 Hz and a politzer bag. The rubber tube running from the bag is placed into the ear and the tuning fork positioned with the stem on the forehead or the tines next to the ear. The politzer bag is squeezed to increase air pressure in the ear canal. In patients with normal hearing or sensorineural hearing loss, increasing the pressure lowers sensitivity to the tone for air and bone conduction. In patients suffering from some sort of stapedial fixation, such as otosclerosis or adhesive otitis media, the sensitivity is lowered for air conduction but unchanged for bone conduction. There are several difficulties to be encountered in the Gelle test, not the least of which is a requirement for much dexterity and expertise on the part of the examiner. The interpretations of tuning-fork tests are summarized in Table 1.

The Pure-Tone Audiometer

Dissatisfaction with the lack of quantitative information provided by tuning-fork tests led to the desire for an instrument that would indicate not only the amount

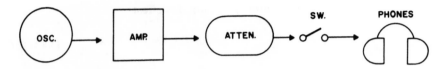

Figure 2.   Simple block diagram of a pure-tone audiometer.

of hearing loss for particular pure-tone frequencies, but the type of loss as well. Such an instrument must be of electronic circuitry with various stages. The first stage must generate a pure tone of desired frequency. This tone is provided by an oscillator that can be tuned to different frequencies. The tone emitted is then fed to an amplifier to increase the intensity of the signal and then to an attenuator to weaken the signal in calibrated units. The unit decided upon for audiometric purposes was the decibel (dB), a unit for expressing the ratio between two sound pressures. After the sound has been attenuated in a calibrated fashion, the signal is fed to an output transducer (earphone or bone-conduction vibrator), which produces the sound heard by a listener. The logical name for an instrument to measure (meter) the hearing (audio) function was the audiometer. A simple block diagram of a pure-tone audiometer may be seen in Figure 2. A photograph of a modern audiometer is shown in Figure 3.

The audiometer was designed to measure a listener's threshold of audibility for various pure-tone stimuli. The concept of *auditory threshold* is currently defined operationally as the intensity at which listeners can just barely detect a tone in a given fraction of trials. This implies that if the tone is near their threshold, they will hear it only approximately 50% of the time. Frequencies originally used corresponded to those of the C scale, and they were even multiples of 128 Hz (low C). In recent years these numbers have been rounded off so that the frequencies found on the audiometer dial are 125, 250, 500, 1000, 2000, 4000, and 8000 Hz. Mid-octave points of 750, 1500, 3000, and 6000 Hz are included on many audiometers, although they are often not tested.

The determination of what was normal hearing or zero-hearing level (HL) for the average normal-hearing listener was largely a matter determined arbitrarily by audiometer manufacturers until the work of Beasley (1938) led to the adoption of the American Standards Association specifications (1951). From this time, zero-hearing level for each frequency was specified with reference to zero dB sound pressure level (SPL). Other specifications, such as the value of the frequency and linearity of the attenuator dial, were also specified. This in effect meant that theoretically the results of a test carefully performed on a listener

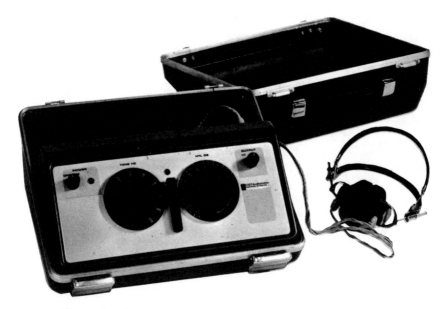

Figure 3. A modern audiometer. Courtesy of Grason-Stadler, Inc.

on one commercially available audiometer would be the same as those using another audiometer of different manufacture.

The adoption of an American standard for audiometers was surely a milestone; however, the disagreement between this standard and those of other countries over what was zero-hearing level for the normal young adult led to the adoption in 1964 of the standards of the International Organization for Standardization (ISO). Since the ISO values were first adopted in the United States, the American National Standards Institute has published a new standard (ANSI–1969). Therefore, at this time, at least theoretically, an audiogram done anywhere in the world on the same subject should yield the same results, assuming that the test is done properly and the instruments are in careful calibration. It must be remembered, of course, that the tolerances prescribed for frequency and intensity are considered by some to be very liberal, which can account for differences between instruments. The SPLs for the ASA, ISO, and ANSI standards of zero HL are shown in Table 2.

The data collected on a listener during pure-tone testing must be done in a very quiet room. The maximum ambient room noise allowable has been specified and can be seen in Table 3.

TABLE 2
Standard Reference Sound Pressure Levels for Zero dB Hearing Level*

Frequency Hz	ASA-1951 W.E. 705A Earphone	ANSI-1969 (ISO-1964) W.E. 705A Earphone	ANSI-1969 (ISO-1964)** TDH-39 Earphone
125	54.5	45.5	45.0
250	39.5	24.5	25.5
500	25.0	11.0	11.5
1000	16.5	6.5	7.0
1500	16.5+	6.5	6.5
2000	17.0	8.5	9.0
3000	16.0+	7.5	10.0
4000	15.0	9.0	9.5
6000	17.5+	8.0	15.5
8000	21.0	9.5	13.0

*According to ASA-1951, ISO-1964, ANSI-1969, and a new proposed standard. Levels shown are those measured in a standard 6 cm³ coupler (NBS 9A).
**ISO-1964 values for TDH-39 earphone were obtained from the loudness-balance data of Cox and Bilger (1960).

The Audiogram

An obvious necessity for examiners performing pure-tone testing is a simple means for recording the data collected on individual listeners. This graph is called the *audiogram,* on which the listener's threshold for pure tones (in decibels) with reference to normal hearing may be recorded for each frequency tested. This gives a viewer at a glance not only the information regarding threshold but, by connecting the points on the graph, a curve that gives an overall impression of the audiometric configuration or hearing level (HL) as a function of frequency.

The audiogram is drawn with frequency (in Hz) on the abscissa and intensity (in dB HL) on the ordinate. The audiogram, unlike other graphs, is drawn with the smallest number near the top. For purposes of uniformity, the distance across for one octave is the same on the chart as the space down for 20 dB

TABLE 3

Maximum Allowable Octave Band and One-Third Octave Band Levels for No Masking above Zero Hearing Level Dial Settings for Audiometers Calibrated to the ANSI-1969 Standard*

Test Frequency (Hz)	125	250	500	750	1000	1500	2000	3000	4000	6000
Air-Conduction (Ears covered)** Octave Band Levels	34.5	23.0	21.5	22.5	29.5	29.0	34.5	39.0	42.0	41.0
One-Third Octave Band Levels	29.5	18.0	16.5	17.5	24.5	24.0	29.5	34.0	37.0	36.0
Bone-Conduction (Ears not covered) Octave Band Levels		18.5	14.5	12.5	14.0	10.5	8.5	8.5	9.0	
One-Third Octave Band Levels		13.5	9.5	7.5	9.0	5.5	3.5	3.5	4.0	

*Levels are in decibels with reference to 20 μPa (ANSI-1977).
**Ears covered with an earphone mounted in an MX-41/AR cushion.

Source: Martin (1986, p. 44).

(ASHA, 1974). Since there is no standard for audiometric worksheets, different clinics evolve their own with appropriate spaces for recording their data in the manner considered most efficient. One such audiogram may be seen in Figure 4. A symbol standing for the air-conduction threshold is drawn at the appropriate ordinate-abscissa intersection indicating the threshold for hearing (in dB) at a given frequency. The recommended symbols are a red circle for the right ear and a blue X for the left ear.

By switching the output of the audiometer, a subject's hearing for bone conduction as well as for air conduction can be tested on an audiometer. This theoretically provides the same information sought on the tuning-fork tests in terms of the air-bone relationship, but in a quantitative fashion.

SPEECH AND HEARING CLINIC : THE UNIVERSITY OF TEXAS AT AUSTIN 78712

AUDIOMETRIC EXAMINATION

Patient's Last Name - First - Middle		Sex	Age	Examiner	Test Reliability	Date	Audiometer

AIR CONDUCTION

Average A C 500-2000			RIGHT								LEFT				
Right	Left	250	500	1000	2000	3000	4000	8000	250	500	1000	2000·	3000	4000	8000
3	2	10	5	0/o	5	O	10	5	5	O	5/5	O	5	O	10

EM Level in Opp. Ear															

BONE CONDUCTION

Average B C 500-2000			RIGHT					FOREHEAD					LEFT			
Right	Left	250	500	1000	2000	4000	250	500	1000	2000	4000	250	500	1000	2000	4000
2	2	5	O	O	5	5						5	5	O	O	O

EM Level in Opp. Ear																

Speech Audiometry

Masking Type		RIGHT				LEFT			
		ST	MCL	Discrimination 1	Discrimination 2	ST	MCL	Discrimination 1	Discrimination 2
AC				List	List			List	List
BC	O		1A SL 30	98 %	SL %			2A SL 30	100 % SL %
Speech									
EM Level in Opp. Ear									

Frequency In Hertz

AUDIOMETRIC WEBER					
250	500	1000	2000	3000	4000

R = Right   M = Middle   L = Left

Figure 4. An audiometric worksheet containing a graph for a pure-tone audiogram. The results of audiometric examination reveal normal hearing for both ears at all frequencies tested.

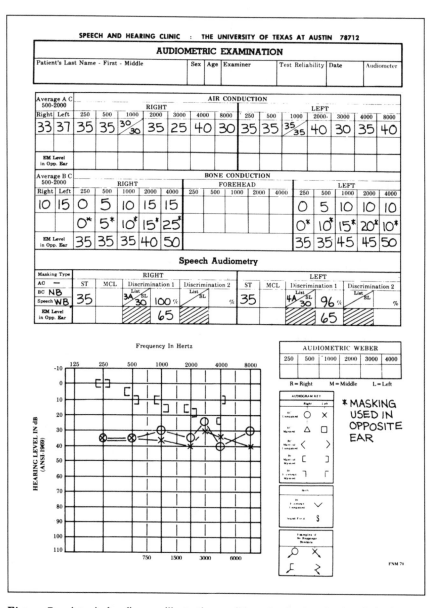

Figure 5. A typical audiogram illustrating a mild conductive hearing loss in both ears. Note that the hearing for air conduction is impaired while that for bone conduction is normal. The speech reception thresholds are in agreement with the pure-tone averages, and the speech discrimination scores are high.

The audiogram in Figure 5 illustrates a person who has normal hearing for bone conduction (indicated by the square brackets pointing to the audiogram's right for the right ear and left for the left ear), but has a loss in the area of 35 dB for air conduction. The loss for air conduction reveals the attenuation imposed upon the entire auditory system by the conductive component, which is shown by the difference at each frequency between the thresholds for air conduction and bone conduction. This difference is called the *air-bone gap*. Figure 6 shows an audiogram very much like the previous one in terms of the amount of hearing loss present; however, the thresholds for air conduction are the same as those for bone conduction. This lack of an air-bone gap tells us that no conductive component exists and that the loss is sensorineural. Figure 7 shows a loss for air conduction of about 70 dB and a loss for bone conduction of 40 dB. This shows us there is a sensorineural component of 40 dB plus an air-bone gap (conductive component) of 30 dB, indicating a mixed hearing loss.

Cross-Hearing

One of the many problems encountered in audiometry is cross-hearing, or *contralateralization*. What this means is that a signal introduced by either an air- or a bone-conduction receiver may be heard by the opposite ear. If one has ever been present in a room in which a severely hard-of-hearing person is being tested, one is aware that sometimes the test signal becomes so loud that it is audible to others in the room before the threshold of the patient is reached. It is obvious that if a patient has one good ear and one bad ear, the tone might be heard by the good ear while the poor ear is being tested. What could result in such cases is a shadow of the better ear, and it is frightening to think of how many misdiagnoses have been made and continue to be made for this reason. A lack of definitive knowledge of the true hearing in one ear, resulting from contralateralization, can lead to an improper hearing-aid fitting, ear surgery, and other consequences.

Many authorities state that the loss of intensity of a sound introduced to one ear but perceived at the other ear averages 50–65 dB for air conduction. The loss of energy of a sound as it travels from one ear across the skull to the other ear is called *interaural attenuation* (IA). Coles and Priede (1968) have shown that the amount of interaural attenuation may vary within subjects as a function of frequency and show a considerable range across subjects. It is obvious from their results that averaging is a rather dangerous thing to do in this instance. A chart of the interaural attenuation for pure tones based on the work of Coles and Priede may be seen in Table 4.

It is generally agreed today that air-conducted stimuli are transmitted to the nontest ear by bone conduction, and arise from the vibrations of the head-

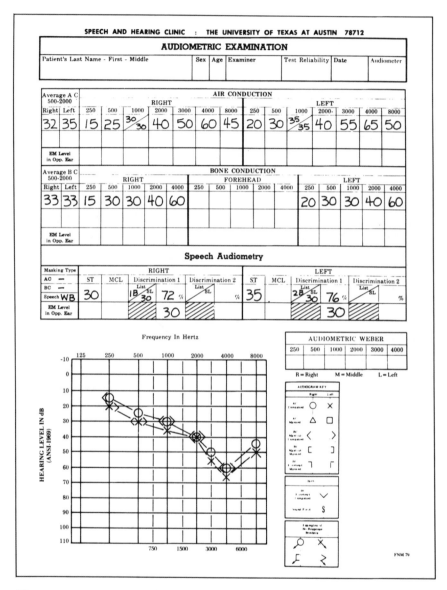

Figure 6. An audiogram illustrating a mild sensorineural hearing loss in both ears. Note that the hearing loss for bone conduction is essentially the same at each frequency as that for air conduction. The speech reception thresholds are in close agreement with the pure-tone averages, and speech discrimination is impaired in both ears.

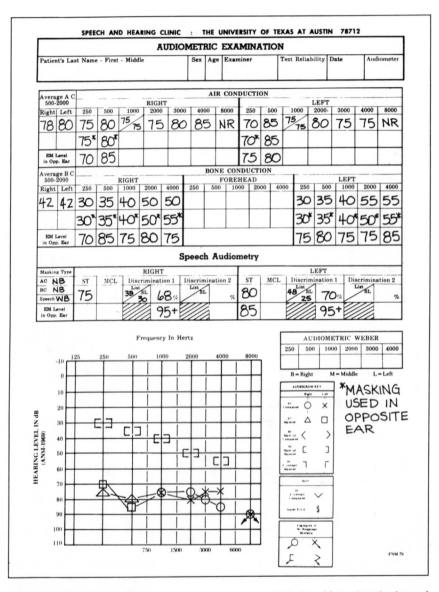

Figure 7. An audiogram illustrating a mixed loss of hearing. Note that the loss of sensitivity for bone conduction is not as great as for air conduction, leaving an air-bone gap (the conductive component of the hearing loss). The speech reception threshold is in close agreement with the pure-tone average and speech discrimination is somewhat impaired.

TABLE 4
Interaural Attenuation (IA) for Pure Tones

Frequency (Hz)	250	500	1000	2000	4000	Average
IA Mean	61	63	63	63	68	63
Range	50–80	45–80	40–80	45–75	50–85	51–70

Source: Coles and Priede (1968, p. 121).

set. Therefore, when deciding whether cross-hearing may have occurred in a given case, a comparison between the air-conduction thresholds of the two ears may not be appropriate. Rather, the air-conduction threshold of the test ear should be compared to the bone-conduction threshold of the nontest ear at each frequency. If that difference is 40 dB or greater (a conservative value for interaural attenuation), cross-hearing may have taken place and masking is needed.

It is now an accepted fact that interaural attenuation for bone conduction is on the order of 0 dB. There are exceptions to this, and there is often some interaural attenuation for the higher frequencies, although this varies considerably from subject to subject.

Masking

The clinical procedure developed to eliminate the nontest ear from participation in the examination involves the introduction of a noise, called a *masker,* to the nontest ear. The procedures for *masking* during clinical audiometry present problems in several dimensions. Undermasking (too little noise in the masked ear) can result in the masked ear hearing tones presented to the test ear. Overmasking (too much noise in the masked ear) results in the noise affecting the test ear via contralateralization of the masking noise. It is not always possible to avoid either undermasking or overmasking, but the alert audiologist should be aware of when they occur.

Masking noises may be of several types, but the two in most common use are white noise (which consists of a wide band of frequencies at intervals of 1 Hz, all with approximately the same intensity) and narrow-band noise (wherein the frequency components of the noise not centered around the test frequency are filtered out). Narrow-band noise has an advantage in that the overall SPL of the noise is lower than if the entire broad band were included, and the effectiveness of masking is not decreased. This means that the noise, while doing as efficient a job, is less loud and discomforting to the subject. Methods for masking reported in the literature vary with the individual author. One area of apparent agreement is that the masking properties of a particular noise should be known before masking can be begun. One way of stating this is to refer to units of effective masking (EM) (Martin, 1967).

The term *effective masking* can be used to mean that whenever a tone presented to the same ear as a noise is just masked out, an effective masking level has been reached. For example, 40 dB of effective masking for a 1000 Hz tone is just enough noise to mask out a tone at this frequency at 40 dB HL in the same ear. This is true whether the subject has normal hearing or any degree of hearing loss up to 40 dB, since any loss would attenuate both the signal and the noise equally. Most audiologists find they must calibrate the levels of effective masking clinically for their different audiometers. This is done by simply introducing a tone, say at 30 dB HL, into the ear of a normal-hearing subject and then presenting a noise into the same ear and increasing its intensity until the tone is no longer heard at 30 dB HL but can be heard at 35 dB HL. This would be 30 dB of effective masking (EM). The audiologist notes the number on the masking hearing level dial that corresponds to this value. Subtracting 30 dB from this level results in 0 dB EM, or just enough noise to mask out a 0 dB tone. Adding 25 dB to the established 30 dB of effective masking is just enough noise to mask out a 55 dB tone. A number of normal-hearing subjects must be used for this procedure. Average values representing 30 dB EM must be taken for all audiometric test frequencies.

A safety factor of about 10 dB should be added to the average value determined to be 0 dB EM to ensure against undermasking in some cases. A correction chart showing the number of decibels to be added to the hearing level dial of the noise channel should be prominently displayed on the audiometer. One way to determine effective masking levels is shown below:

Average hearing level dial setting required to just mask out a tone at 30 dB HL	55 dB
Subtract hearing level dial setting of tone	30 dB
Average hearing level dial setting of masker required to just mask a tone at 0 dB HL	25 dB
Add safety factor	10 dB
Hearing level dial setting of masker adequate to mask most tones at 0 dB HL	35 dB

Sensation Level and Cross-Hearing

In the particular method for masking discussed here, an understanding of the concept of sensation level (SL) is critical. An individual's sensation level for any given frequency is the number of decibels above her or his hearing threshold for that frequency. For example, if a subject has a threshold of 0 dB HL for a 1000 Hz tone and if the tone is introduced at 50 dB HL, the tone has a sensation level of 50 dB, or 50 dB above threshold. If this subject's threshold were changed to 20 dB, a tone of 50 dB HL would have a sensation level of 30 dB, and so forth. If thresholds for pure tones are measured carefully, any threshold measurement, regardless of its hearing level, has a sensation level of 0 dB, since it is zero decibels above threshold. If, for example, a subject has a threshold for a particular frequency of 40 dB HL, 40 dB EM is just enough masking to make the tone inaudible. Any noise that produces a level of effective masking lower than the threshold for the signal to be masked is an insufficient masking level.

According to this definition of sensation level, anytime a threshold is reported for a particular tone, that tone is at 0 dB SL regardless of the setting on the hearing-level dial of the audiometer. In a case where contralateralization is suspected, such as when the left ear is being tested and the right ear may be hearing the tone, the sensation level is known to be 0 dB. What is not known is which ear is responding. If, therefore, an amount of effective masking is introduced to the nontest ear that is equal to the threshold of the tone in the masked (contralateral) ear, only two possibilities exist:

1. If the tone continues to be audible with the nontest ear effectively masked, then the tone must have been heard by the test ear, even without masking.
2. If the tone is no longer audible with masking in the nontest ear, then it was indeed heard by the masked ear initially and is no longer audible due to the fact that the masked ear is not capable of responding to that level of tone.

The procedure recommended here is to introduce to the masked ear a level of effective masking equal to the threshold of the masked ear and retest the tone. It is assumed that all testing has been initially carried out without masking. If the tone remains audible with contralateral masking, then the original result is correct. In cases where no shift in threshold is produced by masking the opposite ear, no further testing for the particular frequency is necessary. If the tone can no longer be heard when noise is introduced, then the masked ear is the one that originally (in the unmasked condition) responded to the tone. If the tone becomes inaudible, then the original threshold was a response from the nontest ear, and it is now necessary to increase the level of the tone until it is audible again in search of the *plateau* (Hood, 1960).

To find the plateau, the level of the signal is raised until the threshold is determined with noise in the opposite ear. Then the level of the noise is increased by 5 dB. If the tone is no longer audible, its level must be raised 5 dB so that the tone may be heard again. These adjustments and measurements must be made continuously until a level is reached where varying the noise intensity over a 10–15 dB range has no effect on the threshold of the tone. At this level, a plateau has been reached and this is the true threshold of the test ear. Noise levels lower than the ones reached have been too low to be effective.

The problem of overmasking occurs when the intensity of the noise in the masked ear is sufficiently great so that it lateralizes to the test ear and produces a threshold shift. Undermasking, therefore, occurs when the noise (directly) and tone (via contralateralization) are both in the masked (nontest) ear; overmasking occurs when the noise (via contralateralization) and tone (directly) are both in the test ear; proper masking is achieved when the noise is in the masked ear and the tone is in the test ear. In some cases, the plateau is narrower than the 10–15 dB range described above, and it is very easy to pass this level without realizing it has been reached. When the plateau is narrow, the situation may change with slight increases in intensity from a case of undermasking to overmasking with the clinician unaware that the plateau has been reached at all.

Masking for Air Conduction

The way to begin masking for air conduction is to introduce into the masked (nontest) ear a level of effective masking for the test frequency that corresponds to the threshold of the nontest ear. For example, if the air-conduction threshold of the masked ear is 40 dB HL at 1000 Hz, the level of effective masking to be applied is 40 dB EM. It should be remembered that a safety factor or "pad" has been previously added to the minimum level of noise required to mask the threshold of a normal-hearing person and is automatically included in all computations of effective masking.

Masking for Bone Conduction

The level of masking for bone conduction is the same as for air conduction, unless the bone-conduction results were originally obtained in the unoccluded (ears uncovered) condition, which is the most popular method. Covering an ear with an audiometer receiver may result in a seeming increase in the loudness of a bone-conducted tone, especially at frequencies of 1000 Hz and below. This is appropriately called the *occlusion effect* (see Table 5). The masking level for bone conduction must be increased anytime the masked ear shows an occlusion effect.

TABLE 5
Average Occlusion Effect Produced by Standard Audiometer Earphones
(TDH-39 Receivers Mounted in MX-41/AR Cushions)

Frequency (Hz)	250	500	1000	2000	4000
Occlusion Effect (dB)	30	20	10	0	0

Source: Elpern and Naunton (1963, p. 379).

Martin, Butler, and Burns (1974) recommend that the occlusion effect be determined for each patient before masking is begun for bone conduction. This is done by measuring the bone conduction thresholds at 250, 500, and 1000 Hz in the normal (unoccluded) condition. Without moving the bone-conduction vibrator, the audiologist places the masking receiver over the nontest ear, and the bone-conduction thresholds are reestablished. The amount by which the intensity required to determine threshold is decreased is the patient's occlusion effect at each frequency. Masking should be carried out immediately, without touching any of the receivers, and the occlusion effect should be added at each frequency to the air-conduction threshold of the masked ear (see Table 6). In cases of moderate to severe air-bone gaps, the initial level of effective masking is often sufficient to produce overmasking.

TABLE 6
Samples of Minimum Levels of Effective Masking (EM) Required for
Masking for Air-Conduction (AC) and Bone-Conduction (BC) Stimuli

Frequency (Hz)	250	500	1000	2000	4000	8000
AC threshold of masked ear	30	35	45	50	50	60
EM level for AC	30	35	45	50	50	60
Patient's occlusion effect	25	15	10			
EM level for BC	55	50	55	50	50	

Audiologists are frequently unable to avoid situations in which minimum masking is at the same time overmasking, as in bilateral conductive hearing loss. They should, however, recognize when this is taking place. Overmasking occurs when the level of effective masking in the masked ear minus the interaural attenuation for the frequency in question is in excess of the bone-conduction threshold for that tone in the test ear. This means that the noise may have lateralized from the masked ear to the test ear in the same way that the test tone may have lateralized from the test ear to the masked ear, probably via bone conduction. Table 6 summarizes the minimum levels of effective masking required for air- and bone-conduction testing.

When retesting pure tones with contralateral masking, it is quite common for thresholds to shift by a small amount when initial findings were not indeed lateralized. This is the result of what has been called *central masking* (Wegel & Lane, 1924). When this occurs, it is quite proper simply to subtract 5 dB from masked threshold results. If the central masking effect is not to have an effect on what is construed as threshold, 5 dB should be subtracted from any threshold obtained in the presence of contralateral masking.

Air Conduction

As stated earlier, the purpose of the air-conduction test is to gain information about the subject's hearing for pure tones as compared to the hearing of normal-hearing subjects at various test frequencies.

Instructions to the Subject

The instructions given to subjects prior to testing can have a profound effect on the test results. Subjects should be told the purpose of the test and instructed to respond to the signal every time they hear it, even if it is very faint. The audiologist should stress listening carefully, but discourage guessing. Directions are usually given to the patient before the earphones are placed over the ears, through a hearing aid if one is worn. At times, in cases of severe hearing loss, instructions are issued through the microphone circuit of the audiometer.

The manner in which the patient responds is largely a matter of the audiologist's personal preference. Many audiometers come with a signal button which, when depressed by the subject, illuminates a light on the control board of the audiometer. The majority of audiologists do not use signal buttons, since many patients become distracted by them, forgetting sometimes to push and other times to release. Furthermore, many clinicians wish to observe the manner in which responses are given in addition to the level on the dial. When a subject raises a hand immediately and assuredly upon introduction of a tone, this may indicate that the signal is clearly above threshold. A more hesitant response may suggest a level considerably softer and closer to threshold. Many clinicians feel that the all-or-none type of response obtained from a light on a board precludes this type of information. For this reason, the response most commonly used is the raising or lowering of a finger or hand. In this procedure the subject is told to raise one hand when the tone is on and lower it when the tone is off. Facial expressions are often felt to be helpful in gauging whether the tone is close to threshold.

Other clinicians prefer a vocal response like "yes" or "now" when the tone is introduced or, for a child, "I hear it." This eliminates much time wasted when the subject fails to lower a hand or release a button when the tone goes off. Some clinicians prefer to have the patient indicate the ear in which the tone was heard, as, for example, raising the right hand when the tone is in the right ear and the left hand when the tone is in the left ear. This has certain advantages when it is not certain whether the responses are valid. However, the additional burden of determining not only whether the tone is audible but also in which ear it is being heard may be too much for some people.

Thus, different methods of obtaining responses are used by different clinicians. It should be borne in mind that the clinician must be alert to the needs of each patient and should modify the methodology accordingly.

Two types of false responses are generally seen in pure-tone testing. The so-called false negative response is the failure of the subject to indicate that the tone was heard. This may occur because subjects are trying either consciously or unconsciously to give the impression of higher thresholds, because they do not understand their responsibility in the test, or occasionally because of loud tinnitus (ringing in the ears).

The false positive response, or response to a signal either below threshold or not introduced at all, may result from too rapid or periodic presentations of the tones, resulting in a rhythm to which the subject responds above threshold and then continues to respond below threshold. It may also result from the introduction of long silent intervals during which the subject feels, "There must have been a tone in there somewhere." There are, of course, occasional patients who try to convince the examiner that their hearing is better than it really is. Thus, the clinician must work rapidly to avoid patient boredom and fatigue, but not so rapidly as to set up a rhythmic or periodic presentation of stimuli.

Method for Air-Conduction Testing

Before testing, the air-conduction earphones are placed carefully over the ears so that the diaphragms of the receivers are directly over the opening into the

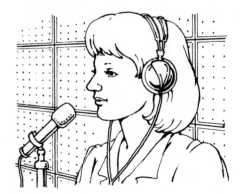

Figure 8.   Subject being tested for air conduction with earphones over both ears.

ear canal as shown in Figure 8. Interfering hair should be pushed aside in positioning the earphones.

The procedure for pure-tone testing as described by Carhart and Jerger (1959) has become widely accepted and practiced. This method has been modified slightly by a committee of the American Speech-Language-Hearing Association, and a new method has been recommended (ASHA, 1978). The new procedure involves introduction of a tone at 30 dB HL. If the subject has normal hearing, a response will be seen at this relatively low level. If there is no response, it is assumed that threshold is higher (poorer) than this, so the level is raised to 50 dB HL. If no response is seen, the level is raised in 10 dB steps until a response is observed or the limit of the audiometer is reached. At each level the tone should be on for a period of 1–2 seconds. Once a response is obtained, the level is decreased by 10 dB, after which 5 dB increments and 10 dB decrements are used. This is the so-called "up 5, down 10" procedure. When at least three of six responses are obtained at the same hearing level, this is considered to be the patient's threshold for the test frequency. In some cases no response is obtained at one level and 100% responses are seen at a level 5 dB higher. In such cases the 50% criterion must obviously be modified. A flowchart illustrating the procedure for pure-tone testing may be seen in Figure 9 (Martin, 1986).

The order in which the test frequencies are tested has not been demonstrated to have any real effect upon threshold. Customarily, however, 1000 Hz is tested first since this tone is easy for most people to hear and has been found

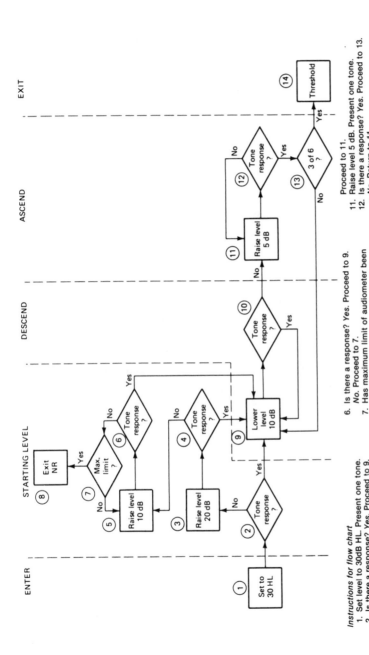

to have high test-retest reliability. After this, the frequencies above 1000 Hz are tested in ascending order; 1000 Hz is retested for validation; and then the frequencies below 1000 Hz are tested in descending order.

The ASHA (1978) method suggests testing the better ear first and then the poorer ear. Any procedure or interpretation based on differences between the ears (such as masking) must be made after the initial testing is completed. There are times, as when testing uncooperative patients such as young children, when procedures should be modified by testing the same frequency (e.g., 1000 Hz) in the right ear and then in the left ear. If only two frequencies are going to be tested during a given session, it is perhaps better to test the same frequency in each ear rather than two frequencies in the same ear. In this way information is gleaned about the relative sensitivity of the two ears, at least for the frequencies tested.

Scoring the Test Results

The results of the air-conduction test are recorded on the audiogram form. The threshold for each frequency by air conduction is shown by placing a red circle at the appropriate ordinate-abscissa intersection for the right ear and a blue X for the left (see Figure 4). It can be seen that the hearing sensitivity at each frequency is well within the limits of normal (no loss greater than 15 dB) in either ear. Since there is no universal audiogram form, the one used for examples in this monograph has been chosen arbitrarily. On this particular form the numbers are written in the appropriate spaces during the test and the audiogram is not plotted until all tests have been completed.

Indications for Masking Air Conduction

Masking for air conduction is indicated whenever the danger of contralateralization exists. This danger presents itself when the threshold difference between the ipsilateral air conduction (test ear) and the contralateral bone conduction (nontest ear) exceeds the normal interaural attenuation for the frequency under test. Normal interaural attenuation as a function of frequency was shown in Table 4. In determining the necessity for masking, one compares not the air-conduction threshold in the test ear with the air-conduction threshold in the nontest ear, but rather the air-conduction threshold in the test ear with the bone-conduction threshold in the nontest ear at the same frequency. Because interaural attenuation values vary, in determining the need to mask, it is best to use 40 dB as the possible IA value.

Masking Method for Air Conduction

As a screening procedure for determining the necessity for masking in a particular case, minimum effective masking is recommended. The method involved is the introduction to the masked ear of a level of effective masking equal to the air-conduction threshold of that ear. The tone is then reapplied to the test ear and the threshold determined. If the threshold remains unchanged in the test ear with minimum masking in the nontest ear, this means that the tone was originally heard in the test ear. The rationale for this is that the nontest ear has been temporarily removed from the test by means of a masking noise and can no longer contribute to the test results. The continued audibility of the test tone at the previously determined hearing level indicates that the tone was initially heard by the test ear. If the tone becomes inaudible with the introduction of minimum masking, it is then necessary to use the masking procedure involved with finding the plateau.

The Plateau

If, with minimum masking, the tone becomes inaudible and the threshold is shifted by more than 5 dB, the plateau method must be employed. With minimum masking in the nontest ear, the level of the tone is raised until the subject indicates that it was heard. The level of the noise is then raised 5 dB. The tone is introduced again at the previously established level. If the tone is not heard at this level, it is raised by 5 dB and then the tone and noise are alternately raised in 5 dB steps until it is possible to raise or lower the intensity of the noise 10–15 dB with no effect on the threshold of the tone. The level of effective masking is noted, and this plateau is considered to be the true threshold of the test ear. Before the amassed results are entered on the audiometric worksheet, 5 dB should be subtracted from the final level obtained to compensate for the central masking phenomenon. A flowchart illustrating the procedure for use of effective masking may be seen in Figure 10 and a diagram of the masking plateau in Figure 11.

Bone Conduction

The purpose of testing bone conduction is to determine the amount of sensorineural sensitivity, or what is sometimes called *cochlear reserve,* for each frequency. As stated earlier, the relationship between air conduction and bone conduction determines the amount of the air-bone gap or the conductive component for each frequency.

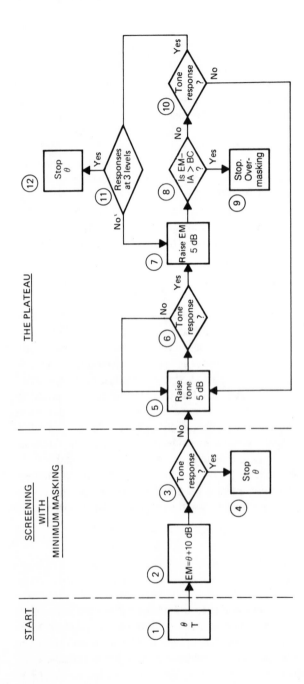

START | SCREENING WITH MINIMUM MASKING | THE PLATEAU

(1) θ T

(2) EM=θ+10 dB

(3) Tone response ? — Yes → (4) Stop θ / No

(5) Raise tone 5 dB

(6) Tone response ? — No / Yes

(7) Raise EM 5 dB

(8) Is EM−IA > BC ? — Yes → (9) Stop. Over-masking / No

(10) Tone response ? — Yes / No

(11) Responses at 3 levels — Yes → (12) Stop θ / No

Instructions for flow chart

1. Start with tone at threshold in test ear.
2. Put EM into nontest ear at threshold level of nontest ear. The additional 10 dB shown in block 2 may be eliminated if that safety factor is included in the original calibration of effective masking.
3. Is there response to the tone? *Yes.* Proceed to 4. *No.* Proceed to 5.
4. Stop! Unmasked threshold is correct.
5. Raise tone 5 dB.
6. Is there response to the tone? *Yes.* Proceed to 7. *No.* Return to 5.
7. Raise EM level 5 dB.
8. Is EM−IA greater than BC of test ear? *Yes.* Proceed to 9. *No.* Proceed to 10.
9. Stop! Overmasking has taken place.
10. Is there response to the tone? *Yes.* Proceed to 11. *No.* Return to 5.
11. Are there responses to the tone at 3 consecutive EM levels? *Yes.* Proceed to 12. *No.* Return to 7.
12. Stop! This is masked threshold.

Figure 10. Flowchart indicating the test procedure for effective masking. From Martin, *Introduction to Audiology*, ©1986, p. 96. Reprinted by permission of Prentice-Hall, Englewood Cliffs, New Jersey.

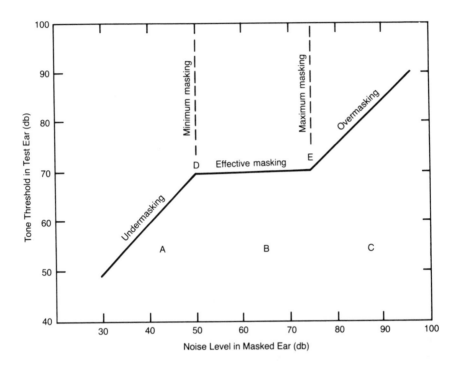

(A) Undermasking. The tone (by cross-hearing) continues to be heard in the masked ear despite the noise, since the tone level is below the threshold of the test ear. *(B) The plateau.* The tone has reached the threshold of the test ear. Therefore, raising the masking level in the masked ear does not shift the threshold of the tone. *(C) Overmasking.* The masking level is so intense that it crosses to the test ear, resulting in continuous shifts in the threshold of the tone with increases in the masking noise. Minimum *(D)* and maximum *(E) masking* are found at either side of the plateau.

Figure 11. The plateau method for masking. From Martin, *Introduction to Audiology,* ©1986, p. 94. Reprinted by permission of Prentice-Hall, Englewood Cliffs, New Jersey.

Bone-conduction audiometry is usually performed by placing the bone-conduction vibrator on the mastoid process of the subject (see Figure 12), holding it in place by use of a steel headband. It has been known for some years that artifacts imposed upon bone-conduction test results are greater on the mastoid process than other areas of the head; for this reason, some audiologists, including this author, prefer the forehead as the site for bone-conduction vibrator placement (see Figure 13). It must be stressed that if an audiometer is calibrated for testing bone conduction from the mastoid, one cannot capri-

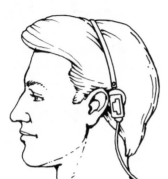

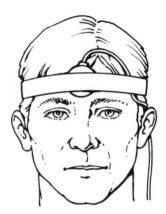

Figure 12. Subject being tested for bone conduction with the vibrator placed on the mastoid process.

Figure 13. Subject being tested for bone conduction with the vibrator placed on the forehead.

ciously switch to the forehead for testing purposes unless the audiometer is recalibrated for forehead testing or appropriate correction factors are applied. The sensitivity for pure tones is approximately 10 dB poorer from the forehead than the mastoid (Studebaker, 1962). However, the advantages significantly outweigh the disadvantages, and forehead testing is superior in many ways.

Instructions to the Subject

When the bone-conduction vibrator is applied to the heads of the subjects, they are advised that the test will follow the identical format of the air-conduction tests. A response is required when a tone is heard, no matter how faintly.

Method for Bone-Conduction Testing

The ASHA (1978) method described above for air conduction is applied during bone-conduction audiometry. If testing is done from the mastoid, at the completion of the test the vibrator is moved from one mastoid process to the other and the test is repeated. If the test is done from the forehead, the testing is accomplished but once. The question of which ear is hearing the tone by bone conduction when testing is done from the forehead is no more germane than it is when testing from the mastoid. The more sensitive ear will respond to a bone-conduction signal regardless of the placement of the vibrator. Frequencies below 250 Hz and above 4000 Hz are not available for testing by bone-conduction on most clinical audiometers. The air-bone relationships at these frequencies must be inferred from test results in the 250–4000 Hz range as well as other audiometric measurements.

The effects of mechanical artifacts upon bone-conduction thresholds are beyond the scope of this book. However, it should be remembered that, especially in cases of conductive hearing loss, the bone-conduction thresholds frequently do not reflect the true sensorineural sensitivity.

Scoring the Test Results

On completion of bone-conduction audiometry, the thresholds are recorded on the audiogram form using a symbol to indicate the threshold for the right or left ear. A key printed on the audiogram form should inform a reader of the meaning of the symbols of the particular audiogram (ASHA, 1974).

Indications for Masking Bone Conduction

As in the case of air conduction, masking for bone conduction is indicated whenever the danger of contralateralization exists. Since for clinical purposes it cannot be assumed that there is any interaural attenuation for bone conduction and that a tone introduced by bone conduction from any spot on the skull will be heard through the more sensitive cochlea, the use of interaural attenuation as a yardstick to measure the necessity to mask is not valid. One should then ask the question whether masking for bone conduction could make a difference in a diagnosis made on the basis of a pure-tone audiogram.

If no air-bone gap exists in the unmasked condition, this suggests either normal hearing or a sensorineural hearing loss. Masking in sensorineural cases showing no air-bone gap contributes no diagnostic information. Since masking cannot improve the bone-conduction thresholds (making the loss appear conductive), the bone-conduction thresholds can only remain the same with contralateral masking, or the noise could cause the bone-conduction thresholds to appear worse than the air-conduction thresholds. This last finding is a somewhat vexing situation that we are sometimes taught should never occur but that is seen frequently in the real world of the audiology clinic and is well explained by Studebaker (1967).

If an air-bone gap does appear in the unmasked bone-conduction results, the clinician must wonder which ear responded to the tone, and the possibility exists that it was not the ear being tested. The resulting conclusion is that masking is required whenever an air-bone gap exists. Therefore, when determining the necessity for masking during bone-conduction audiometry, the audiologist must compare not the test ear to the nontest ear but the air-conduction threshold to the bone-conduction threshold in the same ear at each frequency.

Masking Method for Bone Conduction

The screening procedure using minimum masking as recommended for air conduction is suggested for bone conduction. What is needed is a level of effective masking equal to the air-conduction threshold of the nontest ear, plus the patient's occlusion effect. If the tone can be heard at the same level as the unmasked threshold with this minimum amount of masking in the nontest ear, the original threshold was correct for the test ear. If it cannot be heard at this level, it must be assumed that the nontest ear may have been the one causing the original (unmasked) response. When there is a large air-bone gap in both ears, it is quite easy for overmasking to occur via bone conduction. When it is thought that this may have occurred, the clinician must recognize this fact and note it prominently on the audiogram. Failure to do so can make a conductive or mixed hearing loss resemble a sensorineural loss when masking is used.

The Plateau

The plateau method for bone conduction is identical to that for air conduction. There are instances in which it is not possible to establish a plateau for bone conduction. One such example is the case of asymmetrical conductive loss when all bone-conducted tones are referred to the ear with the larger air-bone gap. In some cases it is simply not possible to assess cochlear reserve with any form of conventional bone conduction and masking.

A summary of various aspects of air- and bone-conduction testing may be seen in Table 7.

Speech Audiometry

The data gleaned from pure-tone testing provide a great deal of diagnostic information. However, in the real world we do not listen to pure tones, and certainly not with any interest in sounds heard at threshold. Therefore, the development of materials to test our hearing for speech was inevitable.

TABLE 7
Summary of Pure-Tone Hearing Tests

	Air Conduction (AC)	Bone Conduction (BC)
Purpose	Pure-tone thresholds.	Sensorineural sensitivity.
When to mask	When difference between ipsilateral AC and contralateral BC exceeds normal IA.	When there is an air-bone gap (more than 10 dB) in test ear.
How to mask	Minimum masking. EM = threshold in nontest ear. If tone not heard, use plateau method.	Same as AC. Add occlusion effect.
When overmasking occurs	When level of EM in masked ear minus IA is greater than BC of test ear at same frequency.	Same as AC.
Interpretation	Audiogram shows amount of hearing loss at each frequency.	Air-bone gap shows amount of conductive impairment (if any).

A *speech audiometer,* an instrument designed to test a subject's hearing and understanding of speech, must first have an input source. This could be a microphone for use with monitored live-voice testing, a phonograph, or a tape recorder for use with previously recorded materials. The level of this input source must be monitored visually on the volume units (VU) meter. A VU meter measures acoustical signal power so that clinicians can monitor the loudness of their voices. From the VU meter the signal is fed to an amplifier capable of raising the signal to a high level (usually 110 dB HL) with a minimum of distortion. This signal then goes to an attenuator (hearing-level dial) capable of decreasing the strength of the signal in calibrated units on the decibel scale to about −10 dB HL. (On the ANSI-1969 scale 0 dB HL for speech is approximately 20 dB SPL.) The signal is then fed to the output of the system, usually one of a matched pair of air-conduction earphones or to a loudspeaker. A block diagram of a speech audiometer may be seen in Figure 14 and a photograph of an actual unit in Figure 15.

Speech audiometry is customarily performed in a two-room sound suite (Figure 16) with the examiner at the controls of the audiometer in one room and the subject in the other room. A microphone and talk-back system are provided for patients so that they may be heard in the control room through the soundproof partition.

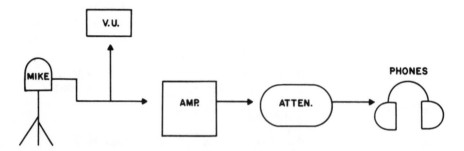

Figure 14.   Simple block diagram of a speech audiometer.

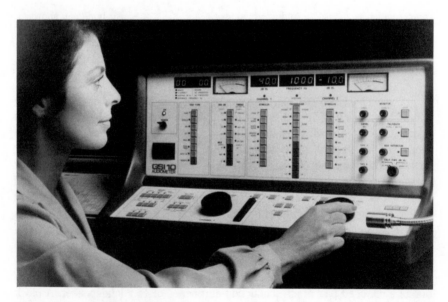

Figure 15.   Commercially available speech and pure-tone audiometer. Courtesy of Grason-Stadler, Inc.

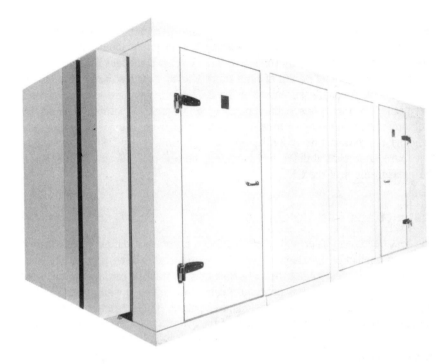

Figure 16. Commercially available prefabricated hearing test suite. Courtesy of Industrial Acoustics Company.

Speech Reception Threshold

It is important to know the subject's threshold for speech. This could be either the threshold of detectability for speech sounds (speech detection threshold) or the threshold for understanding of speech (speech reception threshold). The primary clinical interest has centered around the speech reception threshold (SRT).

There are several ways in which the SRT can be measured. In the method most popular in clinical use in this country, a list of spondaic words is presented to the listener either through an earphone or a loudspeaker. A spondee has two syllables, both of which are said with equal stress (e.g., *baseball, toothbrush, hot dog*). The audiologist must carefully monitor his or her voice so that both syllables of each spondee peak at 0 dB VU. The subject, having been properly instructed, simply listens to the words presented and repeats them. The hearing-level dial is adjusted to the point where only about half the words are understood and correctly repeated. This level is considered the SRT.

For a considerable period of time there was no real standardization of clinical methodology for measurement of the SRT. Some clinicians used an ascending method, some a descending method, and some a method of limits. In addition, the increments of measurement varied from 1 to 5 dB, with most audiologists arbitrarily using 2 dB steps. Chaiklin and Ventry (1964) have shown that there is no clinical difference between the use of 2 dB and 5 dB steps in the measurement of the SRT.

Instructions to the Subject

The test becomes easier and more rapid and accurate if the subjects are permitted to familiarize themselves with the words that will be presented. They may be given the list in alphabetical order or as a stack of cards with one word on each card. Naturally, this procedure cannot be followed with young children or with the visually impaired or language-impaired. The subject is asked to try to repeat each word and is advised that the words will at times be very faint and that close attention is required for the test to be accurate. Guessing should be encouraged. When live-voice testing is used, the words are presented alone. When recordings are used, each spondee is preceded by a carrier phrase like "Say the word _____ ." If the carrier phrase is used, the subject must be advised not to repeat the phrase but only the word that follows it. On some commercially available recordings of spondees the carrier phrase is recorded at a level 10 dB above the test material. This requires a 10 dB subtraction from the obtained results to yield the true SRT.

Test Method for the SRT

The American Speech-Language-Hearing Association has published a recommended method for finding the SRT (ASHA, 1979). The procedure involves 5 dB steps and is basically an ascending approach. The first spondee is presented at −10 dB HL. If no correct response is obtained, the level is raised to 0 dB HL and a different spondee is presented. Increments of 10 dB are used until the first correct response is obtained, after which the level is lowered 15 dB. From this point on, four spondees are presented at each (increasing) 5 dB level. After the patient identifies three of four spondees the level is lowered 10 dB and a second ascending series is begun using four spondees at each level. The threshold is considered to be the level at which at least 50% of the words are identified after at least two series. Figure 17 shows a flowchart illustrating the procedure for testing the speech reception (spondee) threshold, now often referred to as the ST.

Scoring the ST Test Results

The ST, measured in dB HL, is recorded for each ear (and sometimes also binaurally or through a loudspeaker in the sound field) in the appropriate spaces on the audiometric worksheet (see the samples in Figures 4, 5, 6, and 7). It should be noted that the STs for each ear are in close agreement with the pure-tone averages at 500, 1000, and 2000 Hz. A number of methods have been advanced for checking the reliability of the ST by comparing it to the pure-tone air-conduction thresholds. The best method of predicting the ST from the pure-tone average (PTA) is to compute the average based on the best two thresholds obtained at 500, 1000, and 2000 Hz (Siegenthaler, 1964). Unusual audiometric configurations such as a sharply falling audiogram will of course cause exceptions to this rule. In general, the ST-PTA agreement should be within 10 dB, assuming measurement in 5 dB steps or the reliability of either or both tests is in question. Better thresholds for speech than pure tones may suggest a nonorganic component while the reverse suggests a problem in the central auditory system.

Indications for Masking the ST

It is assumed that contralateralization for air-conduction stimuli, including speech, occurs by bone conduction. The danger that a speech reception threshold may have been obtained by signals received at the ear opposite the one under test exists when the ST minus the interaural attenuation is in excess of the best bone-conduction threshold of the opposite ear. The ASHA (1979) guidelines state that a comparison of the ST should be made to the lowest contralateral bone-conduction threshold at 500, 1000, or 2000 Hz. It is suggested that a conservatively low estimate of 40 dB interaural attenuation be used.

Masking Method for the ST

As in masking for pure tones, it is necessary that the masking noise be calibrated in units of effective masking for speech (Martin, 1966). A level of effective masking that is equal to the ST of the nontest ear is then introduced to the nontest ear. An ST is then reestablished in the test ear. If this second ST is the same as the first, then the original results were correct and no further

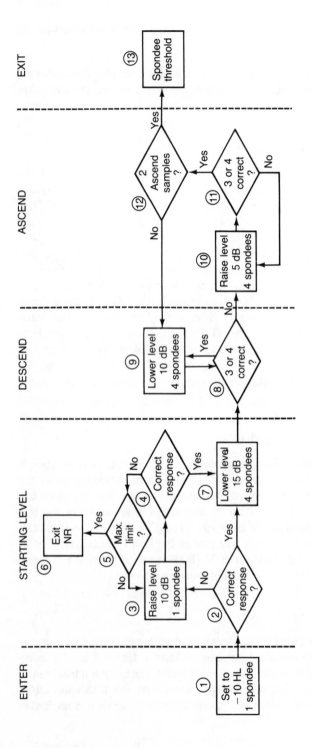

1. Set to –10 dB HL. Present one spondee.
2. Was there a correct response? *Yes.* Proceed to 7. *No.* Proceed to 3.
3. Raise level to 10 dB. Present one spondee.
4. Was there a correct response? *Yes.* Proceed to 7. *No.* Proceed to 5.
5. Has maximum limit of audiometer been reached? *Yes.* Proceed to 6. *No.* Return to 3.
6. Exit. Record "no response."
7. Lower level 15 dB. Present four spondees.
8. Were three or four spondees correctly identified? *Yes.* Proceed to 9. *No.* Proceed to 10.
9. Lower level 10 dB. Present four spondees. Return to 8.
10. Raise level 5 dB. Present four spondees.
11. Were three or four spondees correctly identified? *Yes.* Proceed to 12. *No.* Return to 10.
12. Were 2 ascending samples made with 50% correct response? *Yes.* Proceed to 13. *No.* Return to 9.
13. Exit Record ST.

Figure 17. Flowchart showing procedure for determining spondee threshold. From Martin, *Introduction to Audiology,* ©1986, p. 120. Reprinted by permission of Prentice-Hall, Englewood Cliffs, New Jersey.

masking is necessary. The rationale for this method is that the words in the unmasked condition are heard at 0 dB SL (threshold). If the words continue to be heard with the nontest ear eliminated from the test, they must have been heard initially by the test ear. If the threshold has shifted by more than 5 dB, with this minimum level of masking noise in the opposite ear, the original threshold was incorrect and the plateau method must be used.

The Plateau

With minimum masking in the nontest ear, the level of the words is raised until they are responded to again. Then the level of the noise is raised 5 dB. If the words become inaudible again, the level of the words is raised 5 dB. This is continued until a level for speech is reached that is unaffected by raising or lowering the noise 10 or 15 dB. In recording an ST obtained with contralateral masking, 5 dB is subtracted from that level to account for central masking.

Word Discrimination

It is important in both diagnosis and therapy involving the hearing-impaired to have some measure of the patient's ability to discriminate among the sounds of speech. Such a test must of necessity be performed at some level above the subject's ST since this is not a test of hearing sensitivity. According to Carhart (1965), speech discrimination materials must be (1) nonredundant and therefore monosyllabic and (2) not abstract and therefore not composed of nonsense syllables. There are at present no speech discrimination tests that really meet the desires of all audiologists. What is really wanted is a test to simulate the actual real-life listening situation. Although no such tests exist at this time, many efforts are being made in this direction.

The test in most common use is comprised of 50 monosyllabic words supposedly arranged so that the lists are phonetically balanced. A word list with true phonetic balance would contain a distribution of speech sounds (phonemes) that would be the same as the distribution of these same sounds in connected discourse. With all the possible variations of English phonemes, true phonetic balancing cannot be achieved. The phonetically balanced (PB) word lists are usually delivered by an air-conduction receiver or through a loudspeaker at some level above the previously established ST. These levels vary anywhere from 25 dB above ST to the upper limits of comfortable loudness. Sometimes speech discrimination is tested with PB words at several sensation levels so that a curve can be drawn showing the word discrimination score (WDS) as a function of intensity. In this way one can see which sensation level gives the maximum score (PB Max), or the highest obtainable score regardless of intensity. As a general rule, the initial levels chosen for tests are in the area of 20–50 dB SL.

Instructions to the Subject

Subjects are advised that they will hear a series of one-syllable words preceded by the carrier phrase "You will say _____" or "Say the word _____," and that they are to respond with only the last word of the phrase. Research data (Merrell & Atkinson, 1965), as well as common sense, tell us that responses are most valid when they are written down on a scoring sheet by the subject. This is not always practical, and so in the majority of clinical situations the subject repeats the word.

Test Method for Word Discrimination

The audiometer is adjusted for the proper input signal (tape recorder, phonograph, or microphone for monitored live voice). The gain on the VU meter is adjusted so that the last word of the carrier phrase will peak at 0 dB VU. The words are then uttered with equal effort rather than equal intensity. The output is selected for the right ear, left ear, or loudspeaker for sound field testing. The intensity on the hearing-level dial is adjusted for the appropriate sensation level with regard to the subject's ST. The test is begun, and the subject responds using the method decided upon. Prerecorded materials are obviously preferable for purposes of standardization.

Scoring the Word Discrimination Test Results

At the completion of the test the number of words correctly discriminated is totaled. If the responses were obtained in writing, it is sometimes necessary to check with the subject on difficulties with handwriting or spelling. If the PB words are repeated by the subject, care must be taken to ensure that possible subject speech articulation errors have not had any effect on the scores. The number of words heard correctly is multiplied by 2 and the resulting figure is the percentage correct on the discrimination test (see Figures 4, 5, 6, and 7).

Indications for Masking during Word Discrimination Testing

Whenever masking is necessary for testing the ST, it is automatically necessary for testing speech discrimination in that ear. Since speech discrimination tests are delivered at levels above the ST, the strength of the signal at the ear opposite the test ear is greater than for the spondaic words. It is therefore frequently necessary to mask for speech discrimination when it is not necessary to mask for the ST.

Since lateralization probably occurs via bone conduction, it is necessary to mask for speech discrimination whenever the hearing level of the PB words in the test ear, minus the interaural attenuation for the low-frequency components of speech, is above the bone-conduction thresholds of the opposite ear. Using a conservatively low figure for interaural attenuation of 40 dB, this means that when the level of the PB words (PBHL) minus 40 dB is above the best bone-conduction threshold of the opposite ear, the nontest ear may participate in the test. In such cases masking is necessary to eliminate contamination of the test results by the nontest ear.

Masking Method for Word Discrimination

If the ST has been obtained with masking, then the central masking effect is automatically included in the test results. If masking has not been used for the ST but will be used for word discrimination testing, 5 dB must be added to the hearing-level dial setting for the PB word lists (PBHL) to offset the central masking effect imposed by delivering a noise to the opposite ear. In other words, if the ST in quiet is 25 dB HL, and an SL of 30 dB is desired, the hearing-level dial is set to 60 dB HL. This is arrived at by adding the ST (25 dB) to the desired SL (30 dB) to the central masking effect (5 dB). Not adding the central masking effect could result in a lower sensation level than desired.

To determine the masking levels for word discrimination tests, a formula must be invoked that takes into account the level at which the PB word lists are presented (PBHL), the interaural attenuation (set conservatively at 40 dB), and the air-bone gap of the masked ear. The reason that the air-bone gap is included in the formula is that the strength of the masking noise is attenuated by this amount. The formula for use of effective masking for speech is: $EM = PBHL_{TE} - IA + ABG_{NTE}$. This means that the effective masking level for speech is equal to the hearing level of the PB words (in the test ear) minus 40 dB for interaural attenuation plus the largest air-bone gap (in the nontest ear). A summary of various aspects of speech audiometry may be seen in Table 8.

Immittance Measures

Until less than two decades ago there were only two ways, apart from patient histories, to infer the condition of the human middle ear. One was direct otos-

TABLE 8
Summary of Tests Performed during Speech Audiometry

	Spondee Threshold (ST)	Word Discrimination (WDS)
Purpose	Determine hearing levels for speech. Validate pure-tone results.	Determine discrimination of monosyllables at a given sensation level.
When to mask	When difference between ipsilateral SRT and contralateral BC exceeds IA (40 dB).	When PBHL (test ear) minus IA (40 dB) exceeds best BC threshold of nontest ear.
How to mask	Minimum masking. EM = ST in nontest ear. Plateau if words not heard.	Minimum masking. EM = PBHL − IA + ABG. (PBHL of test ear. IA of 40 dB. ABG of masked ear.)
When overmasking occurs	When level of EM in masked ear minus IA is greater than best BC threshold of test ear.	Same as ST.
Interpretation	Should be +/− 10 dB of pure-tone average except in cases of unusual audiometric configurations.	High scores—normal and conductive loss. Low scores—sensorineural loss.

copic examination of the tympanic membrane to identify abnormalities of its structure or, in the case of its absence, to view directly the middle ear itself. The other assessment technique was by way of audiometry, specifically with reference to the air-bone gap and inferences about conductive hearing loss. The introduction of immittance measures has augmented and at times replaced one or both of these.

With the development of modern electroacoustic devices (see Figure 18) it became possible to determine several aspects of sound in the plane of the tympanic membrane. One aspect is called *impedance,* which in general refers to

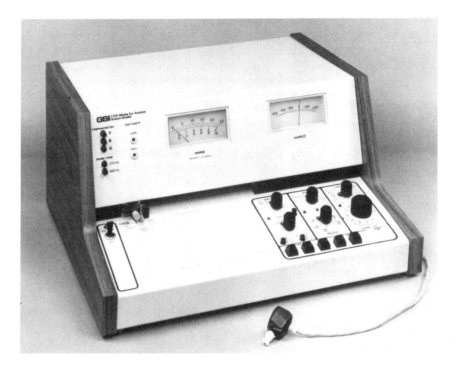

Figure 18.   Commercial electroacoustic immittance meter. Courtesy of Grason-
Stadler, Inc.

the intensity of a sound wave directed at and reflected from the tympanic membrane. Its antithesis is called *admittance,* which refers to sound energy that
passes through the tympanic membrane by virtue of its vibrations into the
middle-ear space. Recently the term *immittance* was coined to signify a com-
bination of both terms.

A diagram of a typical immittance meter is shown in Figure 19. A probe
assembly, which is placed with an air-tight seal into the external auditory canal,
is connected by means of rubber or plastic tubes to one of the following three
major components of the device:

1. A miniature loudspeaker, which is fed by an audio oscillator in the main
   chassis of the device that produces the "probe tone." The frequency of this
   tone is usually 220 Hz, and the output is controlled by a potentiometer,
   which functions basically as a volume control.

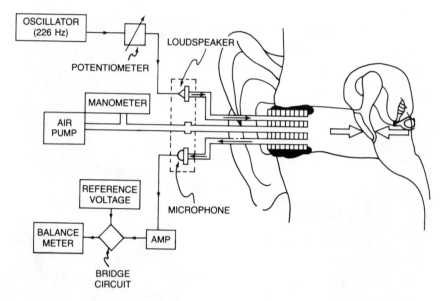

Figure 19.   Diagram of a typical electroacoustic immittance meter. Courtesy of Madsen Electronics.

2. A miniature microphone, which senses the acoustic vibrations emanating from the tympanic membrane (TM), transduces this energy into an electrical voltage and displays the output on a meter.
3. An air pump whose pressure is variable and is displayed on a manometer calibrated in millimeters of water. Pressure on most immittance devices can be varied from +200 to −600 mm H_2O.

When the probe assembly is fitted to an appropriately sized rubber or plastic probe tip and inserted carefully into the external auditory canal, an air-tight seal is obtained. The result is a space that extends from the end of the tip to the tympanic membrane (assuming that it is intact). As the intensity of the probe tone is increased, the overall sound pressure level (SPL) in the cavity is likewise increased, and the microphone senses this SPL until the desired level is reached. The precise size of this cavity is immaterial since a smaller cavity simply requires less intensity of the probe tone and a larger cavity requires greater intensity to achieve the desired effect. Once the seal is achieved and the sound presented, three major measurements may be made: static compliance, tympanometry, and the acoustic reflex.

Static Compliance

This measurement infers the compliance of the tympanic membrane and ossicular chain by comparing the mobility of the membrane under conditions of relative stiffness (partially clamped by air pressure against the tympanic membrane) to its increased mobility when air pressure is equalized on the two sides of the membrane.

Two measurements and a simple arithmetic subtraction procedure are required. First the compliance is measured (in cc) when the tympanic membrane is clamped with +200 mm H_2O pressure (c_1). The pressure is then decreased gradually until the membrane is maximally compliant, and a second measurement is made (c_2). To determine static compliance the following formula is used:

$$c_x = c_x - c_1$$

where c_x is the static compliance of the middle ear. One explanation for this formula is that c_1 represents the compliance of the external auditory canal alone since the middle ear is immobilized. Because the tympanic membrane is relaxed during the c_2 measurement, this shows the compliance of the outer ear canal plus the middle ear. The subtraction of the outer ear compliance leaves the compliance of the middle ear alone.

The theoretical value of static compliance measures is greater than their practical application since modern immittance meters, because of some engineering design limitations, often do not accurately show static compliance of the tympanic membrane. Theoretically patients who show normal static compliance, often considered to be between 0.28 and 2.50 cc (Northern & Grimes, 1978), should have normal middle-ear systems. Those patients showing high compliance (greater than 2.50 cc) would be suspected of having highly mobile middle-ear systems, attributable to such conditions as interruption of the ossicular chain or flaccid tympanic membrane. Individuals with low static compliance would be likely to have conditions of ossicular fixation, such as those caused by otosclerosis, adhesive otitis media, or thickened tympanic membranes. Unfortunately, the overlap often seen in compliance values between normal and pathological ears severely limits accurate determination of the compliance of the middle-ear system in many cases.

Since the c_1 measure is actually one of equivalent volume (requiring more sound energy input to fill a larger space), when that measurement is in excess of 3.00 cc, it may be inferred that the cavity is larger than would be found in even the largest external auditory canal. Such larger c_1 values are prima facie evidence of tympanic membrane perforation, thus connecting the outer and middle ear spaces. Of course, when a perforation is present, the tympanic membrane cannot be clamped by the increase in air pressure, which simply leaks into the middle ear. In some cases the pressure will leak through the eustachian tube into the nasopharynx and no seal is possible.

Tympanometry

Obviously the efficiency of vibration of the tympanic membrane is maximal when air pressure is the same on both sides. When the pressure is greater in either the outer ear canal or the middle-ear space, the tympanic membrane becomes less compliant. Determination of the relative compliance of the tympanic membrane with varying degrees of positive and negative air pressure in the external auditory canal is precisely the purpose of tympanometry.

With the probe assembly sealed in the external auditory canal, the air pressure is increased to 200 mm H_2O. The pressure is then gradually decreased, past 0 mm H_2O (atmospheric pressure) on to −200 mm or even −400 mm H_2O, depending on specific test needs. In a normal tympanic membrane the compliance should be greatest at 0 mm H_2O since normal atmospheric pressure would be expected in both the outer and middle ears. Pressure variations can be made manually with the aid of a dial that controls the air pump, or can be made continuously by means of a motor-driven system. When the manual method is used, discrete steps are employed, often 50 mm H_2O. The results are plotted on a graph called a *tympanogram*. The graph may be drawn automatically by a chart recorder when the motor-driven systems are used.

Tympanograms have been separated into several distinct types by Jerger (1970) for easy interpretation (see Figure 20). It is common for audiologists and otologists to refer to these types, even though there are many patients whose tympanometric curves are not clearly classified.

1. *Type A*. The normal tympanogram is called Type A and is characterized by maximum compliance at or near 0 mm H_2O. This suggests that the middle-ear space is normally aerated and that the tympanic membrane has normal mobility.
2. *Type A_S*. Type A curves are sometimes rather shallow, suggesting that normal middle-ear air pressure is present but that the system is not fully compliant. Stiffening conditions, such as otosclerosis, are suggested with type A_S curves, the S standing for "stiffness."
3. *Type A_D*. At times the tympanogram peaks near 0 mm H_2O, but the peak is very high, suggesting greater than normal compliance of the tympanic membrane. Jerger (1970) called this curve type A_D, the D standing for "discontinuity" of the ossicular chain. Obviously, if the tympanic membrane is not held firmly by the chain of middle-ear bones, it is more susceptible

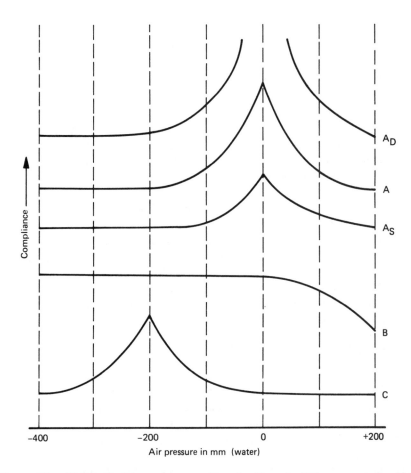

Figure 20. Five "typical" tympanograms. Type A_D. Normal middle-ear pressure; high compliance. Type A. Normal middle-ear pressure; normal compliance. Type A_S. Normal middle-ear pressure; low compliance. Type B. Fluid in middle ear; low compliance. Type C. Negative middle-ear pressure. From Martin, *Introduction to Audiology,* © 1986, p. 183. Reprinted by permission of Prentice-Hall, Englewood Cliffs, New Jersey.

to displacement by positive and negative air pressure. However, type A_D tympanograms have been frequently seen when it is known that the ossicular chain is intact. One possible explanation in such cases is that the membrane is flaccid, often the result of excessive pressure in the outer ear canal (as from scuba diving) or the middle ear (as from excessive nose-blowing or hard sneezing).

4. *Type B.* At times varying the pressure in the external auditory canal does not reveal a point of maximum compliance. In such cases it is likely, assuming appropriate measurement technique, that fluid in the middle ear is preventing membrane motion. Type B tympanograms are therefore often associated with otitis media or serous effusion. There are other causes for type B tympanograms, such as plugged tubes from the immittance meter or a probe pressed against the external auditory canal wall. Type B tympanograms are also seen when the membrane is perforated and the eustachian tube is tightly closed.

5. *Type C.* When the eustachian tube, which connects the middle ear with the nasopharynx, becomes nonfunctional or occluded, oxygen from the outside cannot replace the normally absorbed gases of the middle-ear cavity. In such cases, as the pressure decreases in the middle ear, the middle-ear pressure becomes negative with respect to the pressure in the external auditory canal. That being the case, and observing the rule that the tympanic membrane is maximally compliant when pressure is the same on both sides, maximum compliance is reached when negative pressure is present in the external auditory canal.

Acoustic Reflex Test

There are two muscles in each middle ear, the tensor tympani and the stapedius. Several kinds of stimuli can cause these muscles to contract, but recent information suggests that only the stapedius responds to loud sounds. In the case of normal-hearing individuals the stapedius muscles in both middle ears contract almost simultaneously, even if the stimulating sound is presented to only one ear. This is accomplished by neural connections in the brainstem and constitutes what is called the *acoustic reflex arc.* When the muscles contract, the tympanic membrane is stiffened because the muscle attached to the stapes pulls that tiny bone to the side. The stiffening of the membrane causes an increase in the sound energy that is reflected back into the external ear canal. This sudden increase in the SPL of the probe tone is interpreted as an increase in the stiffness of the tympanic membrane.

The acoustic reflex is usually measured following tympanometry. The air pressure in the external auditory canal is adjusted to the point at which maximum compliance of the tympanic membrane was achieved. Following this, a series of tones at various frequencies is presented, and the examiner observes the immittance device for signs of decreased compliance that immediately follow introduction of the tone.

Acoustic reflexes can be stimulated contralaterally, with the probe tone in one ear and a reflex arousal tone introduced to the opposite ear through an earphone. They can also be stimulated ipsilaterally, with the reflex arousal tone presented through the probe. Ipsilateral acoustic reflex measurements are valuable when contralateral reflexes cannot be obtained in some cases because of abnormal middle-ear conditions or severe hearing loss. In other cases the reflex cannot be measured because of damage to the facial nerve, which carries the impulses from the brainstem to the stapedius muscle. There are times when ipsilateral reflexes are present and one or both contralateral reflexes are absent. In such cases, there is a strong likelihood that a lesion may be present in the area of the brain where the crossover pathways from one hemisphere to the other are found.

As of this writing there is still no resolution to the question of whether it is the loudness of the stimulating tone that produces the acoustic reflex or some aspect of physical or neuroelectrical intensity. It is known that patients with sensorineural hearing loss produced by changes in the cochlea show acoustic reflexes at relatively low sensation levels. For normal-hearing persons the acoustic reflex is generally seen at 85–90 dB above threshold. Acoustic reflexes below 55 dB SL have been associated with cochlear lesions. Acoustic reflexes have been observed as low as 15 dB SL in some cases of cochlear lesion.

In conductive lesions the acoustic reflex threshold is either elevated or absent. In mild losses the intensity must be increased to overcome the hearing loss, and it does not take more than a slight hearing loss before the limit of the audiometric equipment is below the acoustic reflex threshold.

In addition to a loss of hearing sensitivity, any abnormality of the middle ear may make the reading of a reflex impossible. A stapes fixed by otosclerosis, for example, will not yield to the contraction of the stapedius muscle and therefore the ossicular chain will not be pulled and the tympanic membrane not stiffened. This is also true when the middle ear is filled with fluid, because even though the stapedius muscle contracts, the membrane is already immobilized by the fluid pressing against it, and a decrease in compliance is not seen. In cases of interrupted ossicular chain the stapes may be pulled readily to the side by stapedial contraction, but this motion will not be conveyed to stiffen the membrane.

It has been shown (Anderson, Barr, & Wedenberg, 1969) that in cases of lesions of the auditory nerve, such as acoustic tumors, while the stapedial reflex may sometimes be present (it is frequently either elevated or absent in such cases), the muscle relaxes almost immediately following contraction due to the neural lesion. One way to test for this reflex decay is to present the tone at 10 dB above the acoustic reflex thresholds at 500 and 1000 Hz and to maintain the tone for 10 seconds. In normal ears and nonneural lesions the amplitude of the reflex remains relatively unchanged. In lesions of the auditory nerve the amplitude of the response, as read on an immittance meter or by observing the digital read-out in compliance change, decreases to half amplitude in 10 seconds or less. Such findings are positive for retrocochlear lesions.

Examples of immittance measures are shown in Figures 21, 22, and 23. These figures illustrate the theoretical results seen in persons with normal hearing, conductive hearing loss, and sensorineural hearing loss of cochlear origin (illustrated by the audiograms shown in Figures 4, 5, and 6 respectively). There are, of course, many other variations on these results. Theoretical immittance findings are further summarized in Table 9.

Summary

This monograph is intended as an introduction to the basic principles of hearing testing, including pure-tone audiometry, speech audiometry, and immittance measures. There are additional tests which give insights not only into the type and degree of hearing loss but into the probable site of lesion as well. The addition of immittance measures to the basic test battery is useful in this regard.

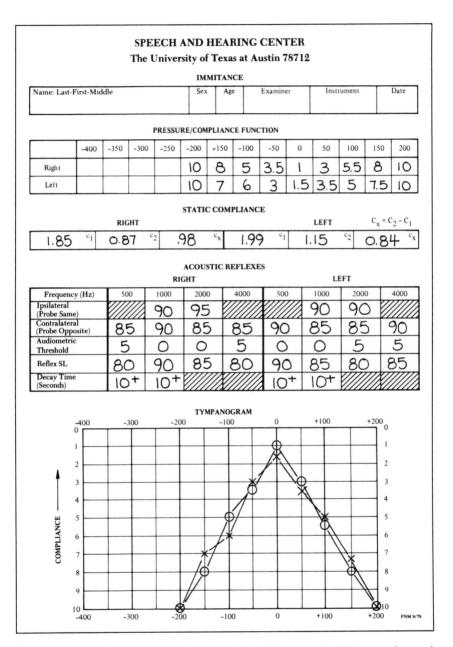

Figure 21. Immittance test results on a patient with a normal middle ear and normal hearing.

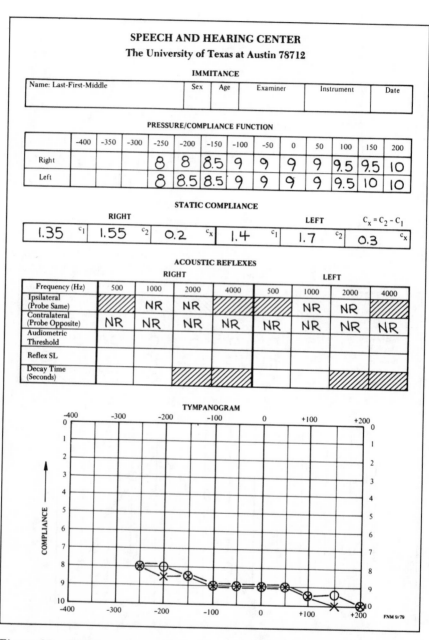

Figure 22.   Immittance test results on a patient with a conductive hearing loss due to otitis media.